Low FODMAP Food Diary

The Low FODMAP Diet has been revolutionary for sufferers of irritable bowel syndrome but keeping track of your daily food intake and deciding what foods are good or bad for yourself during the reintroduction phase can be difficult. This low FODMAP food diary aims to help make following the diet a little easier. For further information on the low FODMAP diet go to www.ibsdiets.org where in-depth food lists and information on the diet can be found.

How to use this diary

Write down the food you consume throughout the day and make a note of any foods or meals that may have caused any symptoms. Under intensity note down the intensity using a scale of 1 to 10 with 1 being no discomfort and 10 being severe discomfort. You may want to make a note of any digestive discomfort, indigestion, flatulence or other digestive problems that the food or meal may have caused under the notes column. After a few days you will be able to start to pinpoint which foods are causing you problems.

Record your fluid intake by marking every new glass you consume. At the end of the day you can put a tick in the stress level box that represents how you felt that day. The bowel movement rating box is where you can record how many movements you have had and what their texture is like - watery, soft, mushy or hard.

At the end of the book there is a table where you can complete a "good food" and "bad food" list when you have figured out which foods are causing problems and which foods you are okay with. This is perfect to fill in when you are on the reintroduction phase of the low FODMAP diet to help you remember which foods you are able to tolerate and which ones cause digestive issues.

Best wishes and good digestive health!

James
www.ibsdiets.org

Date: ....

Meal	Symptoms	Intensity (1 = low, 10 = severe)	Notes
BREAKFAST Time			
LUNCH Time			
DINNER Time			
SNACK Time			

Stress Level (tick)		Bowel Movement Texture and Notes (Watery, soft, mushy, hard)	Fluid Intake Count
🙂			
😐			
😣			

Date: ....

Meal	Symptoms	Intensity (1 = low, 10 = severe)	Notes
BREAKFAST Time			
LUNCH Time			
DINNER Time			
SNACK Time			

Stress Level (tick)		Bowel Movement Texture and Notes (Watery, soft, mushy, hard)	Fluid Intake Count
🙂			
😐			
😣			

Date: ....

Meal	Symptoms	Intensity (1 = low, 10 = severe)	Notes
BREAKFAST Time			
LUNCH Time			
DINNER Time			
SNACK Time			

Stress Level (tick)		Bowel Movement Texture and Notes (Watery, soft, mushy, hard)	Fluid Intake Count
🙂			
😐			
😣			

Date: ....

Meal	Symptoms	Intensity (1 = low, 10 = severe)	Notes
BREAKFAST Time			
LUNCH Time			
DINNER Time			
SNACK Time			

Stress Level (tick)		Bowel Movement Texture and Notes (Watery, soft, mushy, hard)	Fluid Intake Count
🙂			
😐			
😣			

Date: ....

Meal	Symptoms	Intensity (1 = low, 10 = severe)	Notes
BREAKFAST Time			
LUNCH Time			
DINNER Time			
SNACK Time			

Stress Level (tick)	Bowel Movement Texture and Notes (Watery, soft, mushy, hard)	Fluid Intake Count
🙂		
😐		
😣		

Date: ....

Meal	Symptoms	Intensity (1 = low, 10 = severe)	Notes
BREAKFAST Time			
LUNCH Time			
DINNER Time			
SNACK Time			

Stress Level (tick)		Bowel Movement Texture and Notes (Watery, soft, mushy, hard)	Fluid Intake Count
😊			
😐			
😣			

Date: ....

Meal	Symptoms	Intensity (1 = low, 10 = severe)	Notes
BREAKFAST Time			
LUNCH Time			
DINNER Time			
SNACK Time			

Stress Level (tick)		Bowel Movement Texture and Notes (Watery, soft, mushy, hard)	Fluid Intake Count
😊			
😐			
😣			

Date: ....

Meal	Symptoms	Intensity (1 = low, 10 = severe)	Notes
BREAKFAST Time			
LUNCH Time			
DINNER Time			
SNACK Time			

Stress Level (tick)		Bowel Movement Texture and Notes (Watery, soft, mushy, hard)	Fluid Intake Count
🙂			
😐			
😖			

Date: ....

Meal	Symptoms	Intensity (1 = low, 10 = severe)	Notes
BREAKFAST Time			
LUNCH Time			
DINNER Time			
SNACK Time			

Stress Level (tick)		Bowel Movement Texture and Notes (Watery, soft, mushy, hard)	Fluid Intake Count
🙂			
😐			
😣			

Date: ....

Meal	Symptoms	Intensity (1 = low, 10 = severe)	Notes
BREAKFAST Time			
LUNCH Time			
DINNER Time			
SNACK Time			

Stress Level (tick)		Bowel Movement Texture and Notes (Watery, soft, mushy, hard)	Fluid Intake Count
🙂			
😑			
😣			

Date: ....

Meal	Symptoms	Intensity (1 = low, 10 = severe)	Notes
BREAKFAST Time			
LUNCH Time			
DINNER Time			
SNACK Time			

Stress Level (tick)		Bowel Movement Texture and Notes (Watery, soft, mushy, hard)	Fluid Intake Count
🙂			
😐			
😣			

Date: ....

Meal	Symptoms	Intensity (1 = low, 10 = severe)	Notes
BREAKFAST Time			
LUNCH Time			
DINNER Time			
SNACK Time			

Stress Level (tick)		Bowel Movement Texture and Notes (Watery, soft, mushy, hard)	Fluid Intake Count
🙂			
😐			
😣			

Date: ....

Meal	Symptoms	Intensity (1 = low, 10 = severe)	Notes
BREAKFAST Time			
LUNCH Time			
DINNER Time			
SNACK Time			

Stress Level (tick)		Bowel Movement Texture and Notes (Watery, soft, mushy, hard)	Fluid Intake Count

Date: ....

Meal	Symptoms	Intensity (1 = low, 10 = severe)	Notes
BREAKFAST Time			
LUNCH Time			
DINNER Time			
SNACK Time			

Stress Level (tick)		Bowel Movement Texture and Notes (Watery, soft, mushy, hard)	Fluid Intake Count
🙂			
😐			
😣			

Date: ....

Meal	Symptoms	Intensity (1 = low, 10 = severe)	Notes
BREAKFAST Time			
LUNCH Time			
DINNER Time			
SNACK Time			

Stress Level (tick)		Bowel Movement Texture and Notes (Watery, soft, mushy, hard)	Fluid Intake Count
🙂			
😐			
😣			

Date: ....

Meal	Symptoms	Intensity (1 = low, 10 = severe)	Notes
BREAKFAST Time			
LUNCH Time			
DINNER Time			
SNACK Time			

Stress Level (tick)		Bowel Movement Texture and Notes (Watery, soft, mushy, hard)	Fluid Intake Count
🙂			
😐			
😣			

Date: ....

Meal	Symptoms	Intensity (1 = low, 10 = severe)	Notes
BREAKFAST Time			
LUNCH Time			
DINNER Time			
SNACK Time			

Stress Level (tick)		Bowel Movement Texture and Notes (Watery, soft, mushy, hard)	Fluid Intake Count
🙂			
😐			
😣			

Date: ....

Meal	Symptoms	Intensity (1 = low, 10 = severe)	Notes
BREAKFAST Time			
LUNCH Time			
DINNER Time			
SNACK Time			

Stress Level (tick)		Bowel Movement Texture and Notes (Watery, soft, mushy, hard)	Fluid Intake Count
🙂			
😐			
😣			

Date: ....

Meal	Symptoms	Intensity (1 = low, 10 = severe)	Notes
BREAKFAST Time			
LUNCH Time			
DINNER Time			
SNACK Time			

Stress Level (tick)		Bowel Movement Texture and Notes (Watery, soft, mushy, hard)	Fluid Intake Count
🙂			
😐			
😣			

Date: ....

Meal	Symptoms	Intensity (1 = low, 10 = severe)	Notes
BREAKFAST Time			
LUNCH Time			
DINNER Time			
SNACK Time			

Stress Level (tick)		Bowel Movement Texture and Notes (Watery, soft, mushy, hard)	Fluid Intake Count
🙂			
😑			
😣			

Date: ....

Meal	Symptoms	Intensity (1 = low, 10 = severe)	Notes
BREAKFAST Time			
LUNCH Time			
DINNER Time			
SNACK Time			

Stress Level (tick)		Bowel Movement Texture and Notes (Watery, soft, mushy, hard)	Fluid Intake Count
🙂			
😐			
😣			

Date: ....

Meal	Symptoms	Intensity (1 = low, 10 = severe)	Notes
BREAKFAST Time			
LUNCH Time			
DINNER Time			
SNACK Time			

Stress Level (tick)		Bowel Movement Texture and Notes (Watery, soft, mushy, hard)	Fluid Intake Count
🙂			
😐			
😣			

Date: ....

Meal	Symptoms	Intensity (1 = low, 10 = severe)	Notes
BREAKFAST Time			
LUNCH Time			
DINNER Time			
SNACK Time			

Stress Level (tick)		Bowel Movement Texture and Notes (Watery, soft, mushy, hard)	Fluid Intake Count
🙂			
😐			
😣			

Date: ....

Meal	Symptoms	Intensity (1 = low, 10 = severe)	Notes
BREAKFAST Time			
LUNCH Time			
DINNER Time			
SNACK Time			

Stress Level (tick)		Bowel Movement Texture and Notes (Watery, soft, mushy, hard)	Fluid Intake Count
😊			
😑			
😣			

Date: ....

Meal	Symptoms	Intensity (1 = low, 10 = severe)	Notes
BREAKFAST Time			
LUNCH Time			
DINNER Time			
SNACK Time			

Stress Level (tick)		Bowel Movement Texture and Notes (Watery, soft, mushy, hard)	Fluid Intake Count
🙂			
😐			
😣			

Date: ....

Meal	Symptoms	Intensity (1 = low, 10 = severe)	Notes
BREAKFAST Time			
LUNCH Time			
DINNER Time			
SNACK Time			

Stress Level (tick)		Bowel Movement Texture and Notes (Watery, soft, mushy, hard)	Fluid Intake Count
🙂			
😑			
😖			

Date: ....

Meal	Symptoms	Intensity (1 = low, 10 = severe)	Notes
BREAKFAST Time			
LUNCH Time			
DINNER Time			
SNACK Time			

Stress Level (tick)		Bowel Movement Texture and Notes (Watery, soft, mushy, hard)	Fluid Intake Count
🙂			
😐			
😣			

Date: ....

Meal	Symptoms	Intensity (1 = low, 10 = severe)	Notes
BREAKFAST Time			
LUNCH Time			
DINNER Time			
SNACK Time			

Stress Level (tick)		Bowel Movement Texture and Notes (Watery, soft, mushy, hard)	Fluid Intake Count
🙂			
😐			
😣			

Date: ....

Meal	Symptoms	Intensity (1 = low, 10 = severe)	Notes
BREAKFAST Time			
LUNCH Time			
DINNER Time			
SNACK Time			

Stress Level (tick)		Bowel Movement Texture and Notes (Watery, soft, mushy, hard)	Fluid Intake Count
🙂			
😐			
😣			

Date: ....

Meal	Symptoms	Intensity (1 = low, 10 = severe)	Notes
BREAKFAST Time			
LUNCH Time			
DINNER Time			
SNACK Time			

Stress Level (tick)		Bowel Movement Texture and Notes (Watery, soft, mushy, hard)	Fluid Intake Count
🙂			
😑			
😣			

Date: ....

Meal	Symptoms	Intensity (1 = low, 10 = severe)	Notes
BREAKFAST Time			
LUNCH Time			
DINNER Time			
SNACK Time			

Stress Level (tick)		Bowel Movement Texture and Notes (Watery, soft, mushy, hard)	Fluid Intake Count
🙂			
😐			
😣			

Date: ....

Meal	Symptoms	Intensity (1 = low, 10 = severe)	Notes
BREAKFAST Time			
LUNCH Time			
DINNER Time			
SNACK Time			

Stress Level (tick)		Bowel Movement Texture and Notes (Watery, soft, mushy, hard)	Fluid Intake Count
🙂			
😐			
😣			

Date: ....

Meal	Symptoms	Intensity (1 = low, 10 = severe)	Notes
BREAKFAST Time			
LUNCH Time			
DINNER Time			
SNACK Time			

Stress Level (tick)		Bowel Movement Texture and Notes (Watery, soft, mushy, hard)	Fluid Intake Count
🙂			
😑			
😣			

Date: ....

Meal	Symptoms	Intensity (1 = low, 10 = severe)	Notes
BREAKFAST Time			
LUNCH Time			
DINNER Time			
SNACK Time			

Stress Level (tick)		Bowel Movement Texture and Notes (Watery, soft, mushy, hard)	Fluid Intake Count
🙂			
😐			
😖			

Date: ....

Meal	Symptoms	Intensity (1 = low, 10 = severe)	Notes
BREAKFAST Time			
LUNCH Time			
DINNER Time			
SNACK Time			

Stress Level (tick)		Bowel Movement Texture and Notes (Watery, soft, mushy, hard)	Fluid Intake Count
🙂			
😐			
😣			

Date: ....

Meal	Symptoms	Intensity (1 = low, 10 = severe)	Notes
BREAKFAST Time			
LUNCH Time			
DINNER Time			
SNACK Time			

Stress Level (tick)		Bowel Movement Texture and Notes (Watery, soft, mushy, hard)	Fluid Intake Count
🙂			
😐			
😣			

Date: ....

Meal	Symptoms	Intensity (1 = low, 10 = severe)	Notes
BREAKFAST Time			
LUNCH Time			
DINNER Time			
SNACK Time			

Stress Level (tick)		Bowel Movement Texture and Notes (Watery, soft, mushy, hard)	Fluid Intake Count
🙂			
😐			
😣			

Date: ....

Meal	Symptoms	Intensity (1 = low, 10 = severe)	Notes
BREAKFAST Time			
LUNCH Time			
DINNER Time			
SNACK Time			

Stress Level (tick)		Bowel Movement Texture and Notes (Watery, soft, mushy, hard)	Fluid Intake Count
🙂			
😐			
😣			

Date: ....

Meal	Symptoms	Intensity (1 = low, 10 = severe)	Notes
BREAKFAST Time			
LUNCH Time			
DINNER Time			
SNACK Time			

Stress Level (tick)		Bowel Movement Texture and Notes (Watery, soft, mushy, hard)	Fluid Intake Count
🙂			
😑			
😣			

Date: ....

Meal	Symptoms	Intensity (1 = low, 10 = severe)	Notes
BREAKFAST Time			
LUNCH Time			
DINNER Time			
SNACK Time			

Stress Level (tick)		Bowel Movement Texture and Notes (Watery, soft, mushy, hard)	Fluid Intake Count
🙂			
😐			
😣			

Date: ....

Meal	Symptoms	Intensity (1 = low, 10 = severe)	Notes
BREAKFAST Time			
LUNCH Time			
DINNER Time			
SNACK Time			

Stress Level (tick)		Bowel Movement Texture and Notes (Watery, soft, mushy, hard)	Fluid Intake Count
🙂			
😐			
😣			

Date: ....

Meal	Symptoms	Intensity (1 = low, 10 = severe)	Notes
BREAKFAST Time			
LUNCH Time			
DINNER Time			
SNACK Time			

Stress Level (tick)		Bowel Movement Texture and Notes (Watery, soft, mushy, hard)	Fluid Intake Count
😊			
😐			
😣			

Date: ....

Meal	Symptoms	Intensity (1 = low, 10 = severe)	Notes
BREAKFAST Time			
LUNCH Time			
DINNER Time			
SNACK Time			

Stress Level (tick)		Bowel Movement Texture and Notes (Watery, soft, mushy, hard)	Fluid Intake Count
🙂			
😐			
😣			

Date: ....

Meal	Symptoms	Intensity (1 = low, 10 = severe)	Notes
BREAKFAST Time			
LUNCH Time			
DINNER Time			
SNACK Time			

Stress Level (tick)		Bowel Movement Texture and Notes (Watery, soft, mushy, hard)	Fluid Intake Count
🙂			
😐			
😣			

Date: ....

Meal	Symptoms	Intensity (1 = low, 10 = severe)	Notes
BREAKFAST Time			
LUNCH Time			
DINNER Time			
SNACK Time			

Stress Level (tick)		Bowel Movement Texture and Notes (Watery, soft, mushy, hard)	Fluid Intake Count
🙂			
😐			
😣			

Date: ....

Meal	Symptoms	Intensity (1 = low, 10 = severe)	Notes
BREAKFAST Time			
LUNCH Time			
DINNER Time			
SNACK Time			

Stress Level (tick)		Bowel Movement Texture and Notes (Watery, soft, mushy, hard)	Fluid Intake Count
🙂			
😑			
😣			

Date: ....

Meal	Symptoms	Intensity (1 = low, 10 = severe)	Notes
BREAKFAST Time			
LUNCH Time			
DINNER Time			
SNACK Time			

Stress Level (tick)		Bowel Movement Texture and Notes (Watery, soft, mushy, hard)	Fluid Intake Count
🙂			
😐			
😣			

Date: ....

Meal	Symptoms	Intensity (1 = low, 10 = severe)	Notes
BREAKFAST Time			
LUNCH Time			
DINNER Time			
SNACK Time			

Stress Level (tick)		Bowel Movement Texture and Notes (Watery, soft, mushy, hard)	Fluid Intake Count
🙂			
😐			
😣			

Date: ....

Meal	Symptoms	Intensity (1 = low, 10 = severe)	Notes
BREAKFAST Time			
LUNCH Time			
DINNER Time			
SNACK Time			

Stress Level (tick)		Bowel Movement Texture and Notes (Watery, soft, mushy, hard)	Fluid Intake Count
🙂			
😐			
😣			

Date: ....

Meal	Symptoms	Intensity (1 = low, 10 = severe)	Notes
BREAKFAST Time			
LUNCH Time			
DINNER Time			
SNACK Time			

Stress Level (tick)		Bowel Movement Texture and Notes (Watery, soft, mushy, hard)	Fluid Intake Count
🙂			
😐			
😣			

Date: ....

Meal	Symptoms	Intensity (1 = low, 10 = severe)	Notes
BREAKFAST Time			
LUNCH Time			
DINNER Time			
SNACK Time			

Stress Level (tick)		Bowel Movement Texture and Notes (Watery, soft, mushy, hard)	Fluid Intake Count
🙂			
😐			
😖			

Date: ....

Meal	Symptoms	Intensity (1 = low, 10 = severe)	Notes
BREAKFAST Time			
LUNCH Time			
DINNER Time			
SNACK Time			

Stress Level (tick)		Bowel Movement Texture and Notes (Watery, soft, mushy, hard)	Fluid Intake Count
🙂			
😐			
😣			

Date: ....

Meal	Symptoms	Intensity (1 = low, 10 = severe)	Notes
BREAKFAST Time			
LUNCH Time			
DINNER Time			
SNACK Time			

Stress Level (tick)		Bowel Movement Texture and Notes (Watery, soft, mushy, hard)	Fluid Intake Count
🙂			
😐			
😣			

Date: ....

Meal	Symptoms	Intensity (1 = low, 10 = severe)	Notes
BREAKFAST Time			
LUNCH Time			
DINNER Time			
SNACK Time			

Stress Level (tick)		Bowel Movement Texture and Notes (Watery, soft, mushy, hard)	Fluid Intake Count
😊			
😐			
😣			

Date: ....

Meal	Symptoms	Intensity (1 = low, 10 = severe)	Notes
BREAKFAST Time			
LUNCH Time			
DINNER Time			
SNACK Time			

Stress Level (tick)		Bowel Movement Texture and Notes (Watery, soft, mushy, hard)	Fluid Intake Count
🙂			
😐			
😣			

Date: ....

Meal	Symptoms	Intensity (1 = low, 10 = severe)	Notes
BREAKFAST Time			
LUNCH Time			
DINNER Time			
SNACK Time			

Stress Level (tick)		Bowel Movement Texture and Notes (Watery, soft, mushy, hard)	Fluid Intake Count
😊			
😐			
😣			

Date: ....

Meal	Symptoms	Intensity (1 = low, 10 = severe)	Notes
BREAKFAST Time			
LUNCH Time			
DINNER Time			
SNACK Time			

Stress Level (tick)		Bowel Movement Texture and Notes (Watery, soft, mushy, hard)	Fluid Intake Count
🙂			
😐			
😣			

Date: ....

Meal	Symptoms	Intensity (1 = low, 10 = severe)	Notes
BREAKFAST Time			
LUNCH Time			
DINNER Time			
SNACK Time			

Stress Level (tick)		Bowel Movement Texture and Notes (Watery, soft, mushy, hard)	Fluid Intake Count
🙂			
😐			
😖			

Date: ....

Meal	Symptoms	Intensity (1 = low, 10 = severe)	Notes
BREAKFAST Time			
LUNCH Time			
DINNER Time			
SNACK Time			

Stress Level (tick)		Bowel Movement Texture and Notes (Watery, soft, mushy, hard)	Fluid Intake Count
🙂			
😐			
😣			

Date: ....

Meal	Symptoms	Intensity (1 = low, 10 = severe)	Notes
BREAKFAST Time			
LUNCH Time			
DINNER Time			
SNACK Time			

Stress Level (tick)		Bowel Movement Texture and Notes (Watery, soft, mushy, hard)	Fluid Intake Count
🙂			
😐			
😣			

Date: ....

Meal	Symptoms	Intensity (1 = low, 10 = severe)	Notes
BREAKFAST Time			
LUNCH Time			
DINNER Time			
SNACK Time			

Stress Level (tick)		Bowel Movement Texture and Notes (Watery, soft, mushy, hard)	Fluid Intake Count
🙂			
😑			
😣			

Date: ....

Meal	Symptoms	Intensity (1 = low, 10 = severe)	Notes
BREAKFAST Time			
LUNCH Time			
DINNER Time			
SNACK Time			

Stress Level (tick)		Bowel Movement Texture and Notes (Watery, soft, mushy, hard)	Fluid Intake Count
🙂			
😑			
😣			

Date: ....

Meal	Symptoms	Intensity (1 = low, 10 = severe)	Notes
BREAKFAST Time			
LUNCH Time			
DINNER Time			
SNACK Time			

Stress Level (tick)		Bowel Movement Texture and Notes (Watery, soft, mushy, hard)	Fluid Intake Count
😊			
😐			
😣			

Date: ....

Meal	Symptoms	Intensity (1 = low, 10 = severe)	Notes
BREAKFAST Time			
LUNCH Time			
DINNER Time			
SNACK Time			

Stress Level (tick)		Bowel Movement Texture and Notes (Watery, soft, mushy, hard)	Fluid Intake Count
🙂			
😐			
😖			

Date: ....

Meal	Symptoms	Intensity (1 = low, 10 = severe)	Notes
BREAKFAST Time			
LUNCH Time			
DINNER Time			
SNACK Time			

Stress Level (tick)		Bowel Movement Texture and Notes (Watery, soft, mushy, hard)	Fluid Intake Count
🙂			
😐			
😣			

Date: ....

Meal	Symptoms	Intensity (1 = low, 10 = severe)	Notes
BREAKFAST Time			
LUNCH Time			
DINNER Time			
SNACK Time			

Stress Level (tick)		Bowel Movement Texture and Notes (Watery, soft, mushy, hard)	Fluid Intake Count
🙂			
😐			
😣			

Date: ....

Meal	Symptoms	Intensity (1 = low, 10 = severe)	Notes
BREAKFAST Time			
LUNCH Time			
DINNER Time			
SNACK Time			

Stress Level (tick)		Bowel Movement Texture and Notes (Watery, soft, mushy, hard)	Fluid Intake Count
🙂			
😐			
😣			

Date: ....

Meal	Symptoms	Intensity (1 = low, 10 = severe)	Notes
BREAKFAST Time			
LUNCH Time			
DINNER Time			
SNACK Time			

Stress Level (tick)		Bowel Movement Texture and Notes (Watery, soft, mushy, hard)	Fluid Intake Count
🙂			
😐			
😣			

Date: ....

Meal	Symptoms	Intensity (1 = low, 10 = severe)	Notes
BREAKFAST Time			
LUNCH Time			
DINNER Time			
SNACK Time			

Stress Level (tick)		Bowel Movement Texture and Notes (Watery, soft, mushy, hard)	Fluid Intake Count
🙂			
😐			
😖			

Date: ....

Meal	Symptoms	Intensity (1 = low, 10 = severe)	Notes
BREAKFAST Time			
LUNCH Time			
DINNER Time			
SNACK Time			

Stress Level (tick)		Bowel Movement Texture and Notes (Watery, soft, mushy, hard)	Fluid Intake Count
😊			
😐			
😣			

Date: ....

Meal	Symptoms	Intensity (1 = low, 10 = severe)	Notes
BREAKFAST Time			
LUNCH Time			
DINNER Time			
SNACK Time			

Stress Level (tick)		Bowel Movement Texture and Notes (Watery, soft, mushy, hard)	Fluid Intake Count
🙂			
😐			
😣			

Date: ....

Meal	Symptoms	Intensity (1 = low, 10 = severe)	Notes
BREAKFAST Time			
LUNCH Time			
DINNER Time			
SNACK Time			

Stress Level (tick)		Bowel Movement Texture and Notes (Watery, soft, mushy, hard)	Fluid Intake Count
🙂			
😐			
😣			

Date: ....

Meal	Symptoms	Intensity (1 = low, 10 = severe)	Notes
BREAKFAST Time			
LUNCH Time			
DINNER Time			
SNACK Time			

Stress Level (tick)		Bowel Movement Texture and Notes (Watery, soft, mushy, hard)	Fluid Intake Count
🙂			
😐			
😣			

Date: ....

Meal	Symptoms	Intensity (1 = low, 10 = severe)	Notes
BREAKFAST Time			
LUNCH Time			
DINNER Time			
SNACK Time			

Stress Level (tick)		Bowel Movement Texture and Notes (Watery, soft, mushy, hard)	Fluid Intake Count
🙂			
😐			
😣			

Date: ....

Meal	Symptoms	Intensity (1 = low, 10 = severe)	Notes
BREAKFAST Time			
LUNCH Time			
DINNER Time			
SNACK Time			

Stress Level (tick)		Bowel Movement Texture and Notes (Watery, soft, mushy, hard)	Fluid Intake Count
🙂			
😐			
😣			

Date: ....

Meal	Symptoms	Intensity (1 = low, 10 = severe)	Notes
BREAKFAST Time			
LUNCH Time			
DINNER Time			
SNACK Time			

Stress Level (tick)		Bowel Movement Texture and Notes (Watery, soft, mushy, hard)	Fluid Intake Count
🙂			
😐			
😣			

Date: ....

Meal	Symptoms	Intensity (1 = low, 10 = severe)	Notes
BREAKFAST Time			
LUNCH Time			
DINNER Time			
SNACK Time			

Stress Level (tick)		Bowel Movement Texture and Notes (Watery, soft, mushy, hard)	Fluid Intake Count
🙂			
😐			
😣			

Date: ....

Meal	Symptoms	Intensity (1 = low, 10 = severe)	Notes
BREAKFAST Time			
LUNCH Time			
DINNER Time			
SNACK Time			

Stress Level (tick)		Bowel Movement Texture and Notes (Watery, soft, mushy, hard)	Fluid Intake Count
🙂			
😐			
😣			

Date: ....

Meal	Symptoms	Intensity (1 = low, 10 = severe)	Notes
BREAKFAST Time			
LUNCH Time			
DINNER Time			
SNACK Time			

Stress Level (tick)		Bowel Movement Texture and Notes (Watery, soft, mushy, hard)	Fluid Intake Count
😊			
😐			
😣			

Date: ....

Meal	Symptoms	Intensity (1 = low, 10 = severe)	Notes
BREAKFAST Time			
LUNCH Time			
DINNER Time			
SNACK Time			

Stress Level (tick)		Bowel Movement Texture and Notes (Watery, soft, mushy, hard)	Fluid Intake Count
😊			
😑			
😣			

Date: ....

Meal	Symptoms	Intensity (1 = low, 10 = severe)	Notes
BREAKFAST Time			
LUNCH Time			
DINNER Time			
SNACK Time			

Stress Level (tick)		Bowel Movement Texture and Notes (Watery, soft, mushy, hard)	Fluid Intake Count
🙂			
😐			
😣			

Date: ....

Meal	Symptoms	Intensity (1 = low, 10 = severe)	Notes
BREAKFAST Time			
LUNCH Time			
DINNER Time			
SNACK Time			

Stress Level (tick)		Bowel Movement Texture and Notes (Watery, soft, mushy, hard)	Fluid Intake Count
🙂			
😐			
😣			

Date: ....

Meal	Symptoms	Intensity (1 = low, 10 = severe)	Notes
BREAKFAST Time			
LUNCH Time			
DINNER Time			
SNACK Time			

Stress Level (tick)		Bowel Movement Texture and Notes (Watery, soft, mushy, hard)	Fluid Intake Count
😊			
😐			
😣			

Date: ....

Meal	Symptoms	Intensity (1 = low, 10 = severe)	Notes
BREAKFAST Time			
LUNCH Time			
DINNER Time			
SNACK Time			

Stress Level (tick)		Bowel Movement Texture and Notes (Watery, soft, mushy, hard)	Fluid Intake Count
🙂			
😐			
😖			

Date: ....

Meal	Symptoms	Intensity (1 = low, 10 = severe)	Notes
BREAKFAST Time			
LUNCH Time			
DINNER Time			
SNACK Time			

Stress Level (tick)		Bowel Movement Texture and Notes (Watery, soft, mushy, hard)	Fluid Intake Count
😊			
😐			
😖			

Date: ....

Meal	Symptoms	Intensity (1 = low, 10 = severe)	Notes
BREAKFAST Time			
LUNCH Time			
DINNER Time			
SNACK Time			

Stress Level (tick)		Bowel Movement Texture and Notes (Watery, soft, mushy, hard)	Fluid Intake Count
🙂			
😐			
😣			

Date: ....

Meal	Symptoms	Intensity (1 = low, 10 = severe)	Notes
BREAKFAST Time			
LUNCH Time			
DINNER Time			
SNACK Time			

Stress Level (tick)		Bowel Movement Texture and Notes (Watery, soft, mushy, hard)	Fluid Intake Count
🙂			
😐			
😣			

Date: ....

Meal	Symptoms	Intensity (1 = low, 10 = severe)	Notes
BREAKFAST Time			
LUNCH Time			
DINNER Time			
SNACK Time			

Stress Level (tick)		Bowel Movement Texture and Notes (Watery, soft, mushy, hard)	Fluid Intake Count
🙂			
😐			
😣			

Date: ....

Meal	Symptoms	Intensity (1 = low, 10 = severe)	Notes
BREAKFAST Time			
LUNCH Time			
DINNER Time			
SNACK Time			

Stress Level (tick)		Bowel Movement Texture and Notes (Watery, soft, mushy, hard)	Fluid Intake Count
🙂			
😐			
😣			

Date: ....

Meal	Symptoms	Intensity (1 = low, 10 = severe)	Notes
BREAKFAST Time			
LUNCH Time			
DINNER Time			
SNACK Time			

Stress Level (tick)		Bowel Movement Texture and Notes (Watery, soft, mushy, hard)	Fluid Intake Count
🙂			
😑			
😣			

Date: ....

Meal	Symptoms	Intensity (1 = low, 10 = severe)	Notes
BREAKFAST Time			
LUNCH Time			
DINNER Time			
SNACK Time			

Stress Level (tick)		Bowel Movement Texture and Notes (Watery, soft, mushy, hard)	Fluid Intake Count
🙂			
😐			
😣			

Date: ....

Meal	Symptoms	Intensity (1 = low, 10 = severe)	Notes
BREAKFAST Time			
LUNCH Time			
DINNER Time			
SNACK Time			

Stress Level (tick)		Bowel Movement Texture and Notes (Watery, soft, mushy, hard)	Fluid Intake Count
🙂			
😐			
😣			

Date: ....

Meal	Symptoms	Intensity (1 = low, 10 = severe)	Notes
BREAKFAST Time			
LUNCH Time			
DINNER Time			
SNACK Time			

Stress Level (tick)		Bowel Movement Texture and Notes (Watery, soft, mushy, hard)	Fluid Intake Count
🙂			
😐			
😣			

Date: ....

Meal	Symptoms	Intensity (1 = low, 10 = severe)	Notes
BREAKFAST Time			
LUNCH Time			
DINNER Time			
SNACK Time			

Stress Level (tick)		Bowel Movement Texture and Notes (Watery, soft, mushy, hard)	Fluid Intake Count
😊			
😐			
😣			

Date: ....

Meal	Symptoms	Intensity (1 = low, 10 = severe)	Notes
BREAKFAST Time			
LUNCH Time			
DINNER Time			
SNACK Time			

Stress Level (tick)		Bowel Movement Texture and Notes (Watery, soft, mushy, hard)	Fluid Intake Count
🙂			
😐			
😣			

Date: ....

Meal	Symptoms	Intensity (1 = low, 10 = severe)	Notes
BREAKFAST Time			
LUNCH Time			
DINNER Time			
SNACK Time			

Stress Level (tick)		Bowel Movement Texture and Notes (Watery, soft, mushy, hard)	Fluid Intake Count
🙂			
😐			
😣			

Date: ....

Meal	Symptoms	Intensity (1 = low, 10 = severe)	Notes
BREAKFAST Time			
LUNCH Time			
DINNER Time			
SNACK Time			

Stress Level (tick)		Bowel Movement Texture and Notes (Watery, soft, mushy, hard)	Fluid Intake Count
🙂			
😐			
😣			

Date: ....

Meal	Symptoms	Intensity (1 = low, 10 = severe)	Notes
BREAKFAST Time			
LUNCH Time			
DINNER Time			
SNACK Time			

Stress Level (tick)		Bowel Movement Texture and Notes (Watery, soft, mushy, hard)	Fluid Intake Count
🙂			
😐			
😣			

Date: ....

Meal	Symptoms	Intensity (1 = low, 10 = severe)	Notes
BREAKFAST Time			
LUNCH Time			
DINNER Time			
SNACK Time			

Stress Level (tick)		Bowel Movement Texture and Notes (Watery, soft, mushy, hard)	Fluid Intake Count
🙂			
😑			
😣			

Date: ....

Meal	Symptoms	Intensity (1 = low, 10 = severe)	Notes
BREAKFAST Time			
LUNCH Time			
DINNER Time			
SNACK Time			

Stress Level (tick)		Bowel Movement Texture and Notes (Watery, soft, mushy, hard)	Fluid Intake Count
🙂			
😐			
😣			

Date: ....

Meal	Symptoms	Intensity (1 = low, 10 = severe)	Notes
BREAKFAST Time			
LUNCH Time			
DINNER Time			
SNACK Time			

Stress Level (tick)		Bowel Movement Texture and Notes (Watery, soft, mushy, hard)	Fluid Intake Count
🙂			
😐			
😣			

Date: ....

Meal	Symptoms	Intensity (1 = low, 10 = severe)	Notes
BREAKFAST Time			
LUNCH Time			
DINNER Time			
SNACK Time			

Stress Level (tick)		Bowel Movement Texture and Notes (Watery, soft, mushy, hard)	Fluid Intake Count
🙂			
😐			
😣			

Date: ....

Meal	Symptoms	Intensity (1 = low, 10 = severe)	Notes
BREAKFAST Time			
LUNCH Time			
DINNER Time			
SNACK Time			

Stress Level (tick)		Bowel Movement Texture and Notes (Watery, soft, mushy, hard)	Fluid Intake Count
🙂			
😐			
😣			

Date: ....

Meal	Symptoms	Intensity (1 = low, 10 = severe)	Notes
BREAKFAST Time			
LUNCH Time			
DINNER Time			
SNACK Time			

Stress Level (tick)		Bowel Movement Texture and Notes (Watery, soft, mushy, hard)	Fluid Intake Count
🙂			
😐			
😣			

Date: ....

Meal	Symptoms	Intensity (1 = low, 10 = severe)	Notes
BREAKFAST Time			
LUNCH Time			
DINNER Time			
SNACK Time			

Stress Level (tick)		Bowel Movement Texture and Notes (Watery, soft, mushy, hard)	Fluid Intake Count
🙂			
😐			
😣			

Date: ....

Meal	Symptoms	Intensity (1 = low, 10 = severe)	Notes
BREAKFAST

Time | | | |
| LUNCH

Time | | | |
| DINNER

Time | | | |
| SNACK

Time | | | |

Stress Level (tick)		Bowel Movement Texture and Notes (Watery, soft, mushy, hard)	Fluid Intake Count
🙂			
😑			
😣			

Date: ....

Meal	Symptoms	Intensity (1 = low, 10 = severe)	Notes
BREAKFAST Time			
LUNCH Time			
DINNER Time			
SNACK Time			

Stress Level (tick)		Bowel Movement Texture and Notes (Watery, soft, mushy, hard)	Fluid Intake Count
🙂			
😐			
😣			

Date: ....

Meal	Symptoms	Intensity (1 = low, 10 = severe)	Notes
BREAKFAST Time			
LUNCH Time			
DINNER Time			
SNACK Time			

Stress Level (tick)		Bowel Movement Texture and Notes (Watery, soft, mushy, hard)	Fluid Intake Count
🙂			
😐			
😣			

Date: ....

Meal	Symptoms	Intensity (1 = low, 10 = severe)	Notes
BREAKFAST Time			
LUNCH Time			
DINNER Time			
SNACK Time			

Stress Level (tick)		Bowel Movement Texture and Notes (Watery, soft, mushy, hard)	Fluid Intake Count
🙂			
😐			
😣			

Date: ....

Meal	Symptoms	Intensity (1 = low, 10 = severe)	Notes
BREAKFAST Time			
LUNCH Time			
DINNER Time			
SNACK Time			

Stress Level (tick)		Bowel Movement Texture and Notes (Watery, soft, mushy, hard)	Fluid Intake Count
🙂			
😐			
😣			

Good Foods	Bad Foods

Good Foods	Bad Foods

Good Foods	Bad Foods

Good Foods	Bad Foods

Good Foods	Bad Foods

Good Foods	Bad Foods

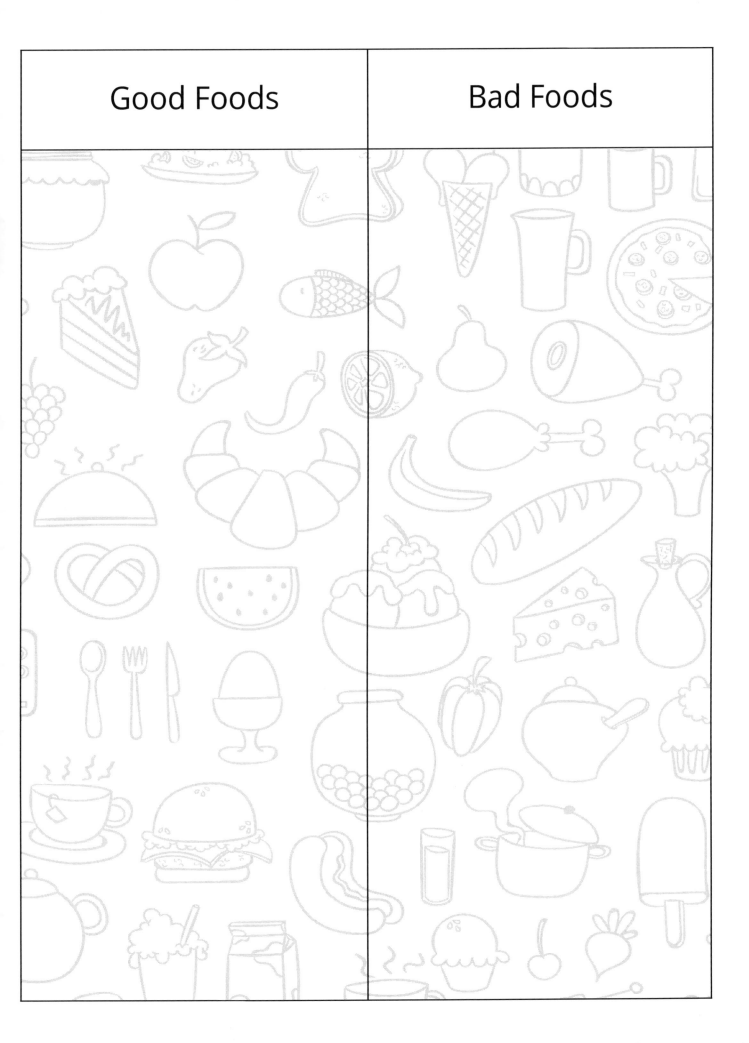